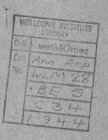

THE CASSEL HOSPITAL FOR FUNCTIONAL NERVOUS DISORDERS

The Medical Director's Report

·I.   ANNUAL   MEDICAL   REVIEW

The Results of Electric Shock Therapy

By Berta Andratschke and C. H. Rogerson.

INTRODUCTION

IN the Annual Report for 1943 a review of modern methods of treatment in psychiatry was undertaken. The value of electric shock therapy was briefly discussed and the indications for its employment were mentioned. In view. of the widespread use of this treatment, together with the controversial opinions which have been expressed concerning its safety and advisability, it seems appropriate to present in detail the results of 3½ years experience at the Cassel Hospital. We are aware that others have had more extensive experience than ourselves ; on the other hand we believe that in our case material is particularly suited for such a presentation. Admissions to the hospital are limited to non-certifiable and on the whole, to recoverable disorders, in which a dangerous and uncertain method of physical treatment would find no place and in which subsequent mental deterioration or other objectionable sequelæ would show very clearly. .

In this report we propose to discuss first the treatment by electric shock therapy of a group of cases which we have termed mild depressive psychosis, since this is the group in which the most effective results have been obtained. We then propose to discuss the use of the treatment in psychoneurotic conditions. Afterwards we shall consider the complications and difficulties which have occurred during the treatment, including in our series for this purpose a group of cases which we have treated as out-patients, but which have not otherwise been as fully studied as our inpatients.

Finally, we shall present a summary of the conclusions which we have reached concerning the indications and contra-indications for the treatment and the results which may be expected.

MILD DEPRESSIVE PSYCHOSIS TREATED BY ELECTRIC SHOCK TREATMENT

In a recent communication (*Brit. Med. J.*, 1st April, 1943, p. 406), we drew attention to a group of cases which we have termed mild depressive psychosis. We pointed out that these cases, including so called endogenous or manic depressive disorders at one end of the scale and exogenous or reactive depression at the other, accounted each year for a great total of sickness and disability. We noted that, since the depression was often masked by physical complaints, anxiety, fatigue, etc., they were often undiagnosed.

We described the natural history of the illness in a group of 100 cases. The essential features were as follows. There was no significant preponderance of one sex ; age distribution covered the whole range from 16 to 70 with a peak in the 50's. The duration of illness before admission ranged from a few weeks to several years. The commonest presenting symtoms were, physical complaints (78 per cent.), depression (58 per cent.), fear, anxiety, agitation (47 per cent.), feeling of inadequacy (45 per cent.). The personality of many had been of the overconscientious, perfectionistic type. A majority had been subjected to some kind of psychological stress, usually for a considerable period before the onset of the illness. In addition 51 per cent. had had one or more previous attacks at some time in their lives, and many showed a family history·of mental disorder of a similar type.

It would not be appropriate, in this place, to enter into a discussion of the differential diagnosis of this illness. Mild depressive psychosis differs only in degree from the more severe depression or melancholia usually requiring mental hospital care. But it is precisely because in its milder form the illness is so common in general practice and so often unrecognised that it is so important. An understanding of its essential character depends upon the understanding of the nature of psychotic depression and how this differs from simple neurotic depression and from the depression of everyday life. Briefly a condition of psychotic depression may be said to have arisen when the individual is depressed without a logical cause based upon his relationship with external reality, or when his state of depression is grossly disproportionate to the cause or persists unduly after the removal of the cause. In ungraceful but expressive terms he has become " stuck " in a state of depression and *his mood governs his view of external reality.* In " normal " situational depression on the other hand such as that which occurs after bereavement or bad news *his view of external reality governs his mood.* ,

Neurotic depression is closely akin to " normal " situational depression in that the same cause and effect relationship to external reality is preserved. The depression may appear disproportionate to its cause as judged by the casual observer, but in the light of its significance to the psychoneurotic patient the cause is present and it is adequate.

The whole of this group whose treatment is about to be described was considered by us to be suffering from a condition of psychotic depression.

The Technique of Treatment

The patient is given a light breakfast at 7.30 a.m., the treatment is given at about 11 a.m. The apparatus used is made by the Solus Company. The patient is placed upon a rigid mattress with a rolled up blanket under his thoracic spine. A specially constructed rubber gag is placed between the teeth and firm pressure is applied to the shoulders, hips and lower jaw. Support to the jaw greatly reduces the risk of dislocation. The extension of the spine almost completely abolishes serious complaints of backache after treatment and seems to have eliminated crush fractures of the bodies of one or more vertebrae which was at one time a fairly common radiological finding in the experience of many workers.

Standard electrodes are applied to the fronto-parietal region, using a diathermy contact paste. The initial dosage is usually 130 volts for 0.3 seconds. If no convulsion occurs the dose is raised to 150 volts, and if necessary to 0.5 seconds. In our experience it is useless or even harmful to give a sub-convulsive dose. If this maximum time and voltage are ineffective they can usually be rendered adequate by previous hyper-ventilation. Cyanosis often occurs at the end of the convulsion ; it is treated by administration of oxygen through a nasal catheter. It has seldom given cause for anxiety.

Excessive salivation can be checked by giving atropine or belladonna before treatment. We use,

as a routine, a pill containing extract belladonna siccum gr. ¼. Sodium amytal in 3 or 6 grain doses serves a useful purpose to allay apprehension in nervous patients. It is also said to " soften " the convulsion slightly. It does not appear to raise the convulsive threshold to any serious degree. Phenobarbitone on the other hand certainly has this effect and is avoided during treatment.

Results

A study of the natural history of this disorder reveals that the majority of cases recover spontaneously. There is, however, an extraordinary variability in the duration of the attack which may last from a few weeks or even days to many years. The use of electric shock therapy cannot therefore be justified simply by a presentation of recovery rates. The important feature of the treatment is that recovery occurs as an immediate and usually predictable sequel with an immense saving of hospital time, personal misery and social disturbance. It is probable that the final recovery rate with shock therapy is higher than without it, since, in chronic depression, rut formation and lasting invalidism, are common. There is also likely to be a considerable reduction in the suicide rate. Both these points are at present difficult to demonstrate but the shortening of the duration of the illness and the consequent lessening of its seriousness is vividly demonstrated by our case material. Since October, 1941, we have discharged 72 patients suffering from mild depressive psychosis who have been treated with electric shock therapy. We have used the treatment as a routine in all cases in which spontaneous recovery does not appear likely to occur within a few weeks of admission to hospital. We base our judgment on various factors, including the known duration of previous attacks, the duration of the present illness, and the immediate response of the illness to routine hospital treatment. Special contra-indications will be mentioned below. Results are shown in Table 1.

TABLE I

Results of Electric Shock Therapy
72 Cases of Mild Depressive Psychosis

Much Improved*	Improved	Not Improved	Total
54	12	6	72
Percentage 75%	17%	8%	100%

Mean duration of stay in hospital—13 weeks (approx.).

* "Much improved" includes those patients who have lost all symptoms of mental disorder and those in whom only such minor psychopathic traits persist as will not seriously interfere with their adjustment to normal life.

2

The mean duration of stay in hospital included preliminary investigations and a subsequent period of psychotherapy, which we consider essential. The average number of treatments administered for each patient in the whole group was 7.8.

Nature of Control Group

In contrasting these results with those which were obtained in cases of depression before shock therapy was instituted, it is necessary to bear in mind that the Cassel Hospital has not been in a position to accept for treatment patients likely to prove chronic, or inaccessible to treatment, or suicidal. Many cases of depression had therefore formerly to be discharged unimproved because they were not considered suitable for retention in the hospital. Some of these were referred to mental hospital, others returned home. The 75 patients in the control group represent the cases of mild depressive psychoses which were actually retained for treatment during the years 1938 and 1939. These are a more carefully selected, more favourable group than the shock therapy series. Results are shown in Table 2.

TABLE 2

75 Selected Cases of Depression Treated Without Shock Therapy

Much Improved	Improved	Not Improved	Total
40	19	16	75
Percentage 53.3%	25.3%	21.4%	100%

Mean duration of stay in hospital—26 weeks (approx.)

CONCLUSION

The conclusion which appears inescapable is that the use of electric shock therapy has rendered depressive psychosis a much less devastating disorder than formerly. It now responds to active treatment rather than to custodial care, with all the difference in outlook which that change implies. It appears equally obvious that unless there is a definite incidence of serious complications, the question must be not whether the treatment should be administered but whether in a given case there is any legitimate reason for withholding it.

COMMENT

The rapid recovery rate in states of depression treated by electric shock treatment is so high that the few complete or partial failures occurring become rather conspicuous.

A survey of these cases (18 in all) shows that definite factors played a part in the unsatisfactory response to the treatment.

In six patients the selective influence of electric shock treatment on the depressive element in the illness was clearly shown. It was equally clear that other underlying difficulties were but little influenced. Three of the six showed a life-long background of maladjustment in a psychopathic direction (alcoholism, homosexuality) and three an admixture of schizoid reactions. Two of these patients were later admitted to mental hospitals with a diagnosis of schizophrenia. On admission the depression was the most outstanding element and had overshadowed the underlying grave personality disorder. It is not surprising that shock treatment did not have a permanent or complete effect.

In a group of six patients the treatment had to be prematurely interrupted. On four occasions this was due to the development of confusional states which will be further discussed under the heading of "Complications." One patient refused further treatment after she had had three and in one case rising blood pressure prevented further treatment.

Three patients showed a very satisfactory response to treatment—the depression disappeared—but these three patients had to leave for domestic reasons immediately after the treatment was completed and before a proper psychological approach had been possible; we therefore did not feel justified in classifying these patients as much improved.

In the remaining three patients there were none of these factors—no serious underlying personality disorder, no premature interruption of treatment, no premature discharge from hospital—and yet no response to the treatment. It is interesting to note that two out of these three were true manic depressives who had had in the past a number of both depressive and manic episodes. Both had once benefited by shock treatment—but failed to benefit by it a second time.

The last of these presented a typical recurrent depression without manic episodes. Personality, between attacks was well preserved and no explanation can be offered for the failure of treatment in this case.

3

SHOCK THERAPY IN TREATMENT OF NEUROSIS

Thirty in-patients suffering from neurosis have received shock therapy. It is impossible to present the results in a form as clear-cut as for the depressive group. In the first place this is a heterogeneous series with a small number of cases of each type compared to the relative homogeneity of the depressive group. In the second place recovery did not usually occur as a rapid and immediate sequel to the treatment as in the case of the depressions. In this series the treatment was applied either as a last hope in a difficult case or as an attempt to break up a chronic anxiety state or obsessional neurosis. It then became one step in a series of efforts each one of which may have contributed a substantial part to the final result.

The results are shown in the table.

Electric Shock Therapy
Results of Treatment in Thirty Cases of Neurosis

Diagnosis	No. of Cases	Much Improved	Improved	Not Improved
Anxiety neurosis	16	7	7	2
Obsessional neurosis	3	0	3	0
Hysteria	7	2	2	3
Unclassified	4	2	1	1
Total Neurosis	30	11	13	6
Percentage	100%	37%	43%	20%

This table presents a marked contrast to the table showing the results of treatment of the depressions. Since it is not claimed that shock therapy was the only, or indeed necessarily the major factor in recovery of this series, the question arises whether the treatment is justified at all in the neuroses. As the numbers are so small it is better to attempt to answer it by a clinical survey of the individual groups.

(1) *Affective neurosis (anxiety neurosis)*. Here seven patients were much improved, seven patients improved and two not improved. All of these patients were suffering from chronic anxiety states of long duration. The treatment was administered because intensive psychotherapy or other forms of physical treatment had failed to break up the anxiety state. We believe that the final result was definitely more satisfactory in the majority of them than it would otherwise have been. We are profoundly conscious that shock therapy can never be a substitute for psychotherapy in such cases. It is indeed absurd to suppose that difficult life situations and complex determined ideas can be eliminated by the passage of an electrical current. But patterns of behaviour may become chronic and impossible to modify psychotherapeutically even though their nature may be appreciated by doctor and patient alike. It is in the face of this occurrence that shock therapy may be of use. It must be administered after careful weighing up of all the factors in a given case and as part of a general plan of treatment. We believe that, contrary to the opinion of some, its use may then in certain cases be justified.

(2) *Obsessional Neurosis*. In this very small group three cases showed some improvement. It must be emphasised that obsessional symptoms often occur in the course of a depressive psychosis. Such cases have in our series been grouped among the depressions where they properly belong. The three cases in this series were all disappointing as their initial response to treatment was good. However, unfortunately, they relapsed soon after the conclusion of the treatment. We are now proposing to try the effect of a " maintenance dose " of treatment about once a fortnight for a considerable period in the hope of producing more permanent results. The treatment by psychotherapy of severe obsessional neuroses is difficult and often unsatisfactory. The operation of pre-frontal leucotomy has proved helpful, but, we do not yet think that it can be recommended in any but incapacitating illnesses. There remain those cases in which there is not total incapacity, in which in fact work may be performed

of a highly skilled nature but in which life may nevertheless be rendered miserable by obsessional symptoms. For these cases a successful technique of treatment by electric shock therapy would be a most valuable achievement.

(3) *Hysteria.* We have treated seven cases of conversion hysteria by means of shock therapy. We do not believe that they derived much benefit from the treatment and we have abandoned its use in this condition.

(4) *Unclassified Neurosis.* This group, representing mainly chronic psychopathic personality disorders with inadequacy and depression, is too small to justify comment.

COMPLICATIONS

Before describing the complications which have occurred during treatment it is necessary to bring into the picture certain other cases.

Three patients suffering from schizophrenic reactions have been treated during the period under review. None of these patients improved except temporarily. Few schizophrenic disorders are admitted to the hospital and it has become our custom to refer all of them elsewhere for full insulin coma therapy if possible.

Twenty-seven outpatients received treatment, 15 men and 12 women. The majority of these patients were suffering from depression. Nearly all of them were referred by outside psychiatrists and were returned to their own psychiatrist when treatment was completed. Thus we have not the same detailed information about them as about our own in-patients and we have not included them in our detailed discussion of results.

We have, however, been able to ascertain that the group as a whole has shown satisfactory results, and we have observed the incidence of complications with especial care.

The conclusion we have reached is that although we prefer to have the patient in hospital for treatment, there is no inherent reason why outpatient treatment should not be undertaken. Co-operative relatives, adequate supervision at home and facilities for immediate admission to hospital in case of need are all essential. It is obvious that if the chief precipitating factors in the illness are to be found at home, hospitalisation is necessary.

Taking all these cases into consideration we are in a position to survey the complications which have arisen during the treatment of 132 patients.

Complications of Treatment

The complications may be divided into :

(a) Very mild complications, so mild in fact that they could be termed accompanying

symptoms of shock treatment rather than complications.

(b) More serious complications.

A. Accompanying Symptoms

(1) *Physical.* Pain in the back was a very common complaint before we employed a rigid mattress with a rolled up blanket under the thoracic spine with pressure on shoulders and hips to prevent flexion of the spine. Since then we hear occasionally complaints of pains in the back or in various groups of muscles related to the severity of the convulsions. Massage after treatment, which is carried out as a matter of routine in every case, greatly relieves these pains.

Partial dislocation of the jaw was common before our technique was improved—it has never presented a real clinical problem. With skilled nursing assistance it is now very rare.

(2) *Psychological.* There is frequently some amnesia for the period immediately preceding the treatment. Sometimes there is a more extensive amnesia of a patchy character involving events which have occurred during the previous few months. There is a special tendency to forget proper names, and there is some difficulty with regard to recent memory. This impairment of memory varies greatly from patient to patient and is not dependent on age or intellectual capacity. We have noticed that patients who know something of the possible after effects of this treatment complain much more of forgetfulness than others who have no knowledge of it.

In no case has any series defect persisted beyond a month after shock treatment was concluded.

Recovery from depression, following shock therapy is sometimes accompanied by very mild elation and push of activity. Whether such trivial elation occurs with equal frequency after spontaneous recovery we are not in a position to say. We have never previously observed, in so short a time, so many satisfactory recoveries from depression.

B. Complications

(1) *Physical.* Three cases of fractures were found. Two showed partial crush fractures of two thoracic vertebræ (these incidents occurred in the beginning of our series). Another patient suffered a fracture of the scapula. This patient had a marked Kyphoscoliosis. It should be noted that we have not made routine X-rays of the spine of all patients. This has only been done when complaint of pain and stiffness would appear to warrant it.

Damage to teeth is likely to occur if a hard cored gag is used (e.g. a wooden spatula covered with lint). In the absence of obvious trauma periodontitis has also occurred in teeth especially subject to pressure. We are informed by our consulting dental

5

surgeon Mr. Myatt that serious devitalisation of teeth may result and may not be apparent for several months. In collaboration with him a special gag has been devised which has largely overcome this difficulty. It also provides a convenient airway through which oxygen may be administered if marked cyanosis occurs.

(2) *Psychological.* There is a condition of a more serious nature but still of a transitory character which we have termed excitement with confusion. It occurred in seven patients in our series, six females aged between 38 and 55 and one male aged 40. Four of these have not been straightforward, uncomplicated depressive states, but presented an admixture of paranoid or hysterical features.

Without any warning usually after four or five treatments and within a few hours of the most recent one the patient becomes disorientated, restless, confused and excited. He may show evidence of auditory or visual hallucinations.

The reaction appears to be a benign and short-lived one, but the patients present an acute nursing problem. They may refuse food and sedatives and require constant supervision. Owing to the difficulty involved in keeping them in a neurosis unit the first two were transferred to a mental hospital as temporary patients. In later cases it was found that there was a rapid response to continuous narcosis therapy combined with large doses of Vitamin B. All seven patients recovered within two weeks without evidence of subsequent mental impairment.

In addition to these, one patient, a male aged 52, developed paranoid symptoms after 10 treatments, though he had recovered completely from his depression. Later investigation revealed that he had shown mild paranoid symptoms during a previous attack of depression.

One patient, a female aged 44, jumped out of the window one night after four treatments. This was done with no suicidal intentions ; she threw her eiderdown out first. She was not seriously confused but acted rather on impulse ; she stated she wanted to go home just then. This patient had shown paranoid tendencies before her depressive illness.

Both these patients subsequently improved.

It is impossible to predict which patient might react with a confusional state to the treatment, so that the possible occurrence of such incidents calls for care in administering the treatment to out-patients. Away from hospital it would be both dangerous and frightening to relatives. In our opinion out-patient treatment should always be backed by facilities for immediate admission to hospital if needed.

Summary

The above incidence of serious complications, namely, three known fractures, none producing any permanent disability, seven temporary states of confusion and two paranoid outbursts in previously paranoid personalities, out of a total of 132 patients treated, demand that the treatment should be administered with care and forethought. They do not, in our opinion, contra indicate its use in the painful and distressing disorders for which it is beneficial.

FINAL CONCLUSION

Electric shock therapy is capable of terminating a depressive psychosis in a very large majority of cases. It will fail to be effective if factors in the personality are heavily weighted against recovery. It would perhaps be true to say that those patients who might eventually recover in any case will recover quickly under shock therapy. The final recovery rates will, however, be better than that in any control series, since suicide, death from inter-current illness and chronic invalidism will all take their toll in such a long unhappy illness.

The complications of the treatment are not such as to justify withholding it in any case where spontaneous recovery does not seem imminent.

The treatment is of some assistance in cases of chronic anxiety neurosis, but here it should only be used after particularly careful consideration.

In our small experience it has proved disappointing for obsessional states and for other forms of neurosis.

We have no experience of its use in manic states and not enough to justify comment in schizophrenic states.

List of Publications during 1944 :

ROGERSON, C. H. : " Narco-Analysis with Nitrous Oxide," *Brit. Med. J.* Volume I, page 811, June.

ROGERSON, C. H. and HANN, Miss O. P. E. (Matron) : " Post Graduate Training in Psychiatry," *Nursing Mirror*, September.

NURSING

Members of nursing staff holding Cassel Hospital Certificates :—

     Miss O. P. E. HANN, S.R.N., D.N. (*Matron*).

     Miss J. EVANS, S.R.N. (*Assistant Matron*).

     Miss E. NETTLESHIP, S.R.N.

     Miss F. WADDINGTON, S.R.N.

     Miss R. BRIDGE, S.R.N.

     Miss M. METCALFE, S.R.N.

The outstanding event of the year was the presentation of certificates and prizes to those members of the nursing staff who had completed the full course of training at the hospital. This took place in May, the presentations being made by Air-Commodore R. D. Gillespie, who spoke about the work of the hospital and the importance of psychiatric nursing.

The prize-giving was followed by lectures and demonstrations of psychiatric work which evoked great interest among the professional and non-professional groups present. The success of these demonstrations was such that the introduction of short intensive courses is being considered.

There are signs of steadily increasing interest in psychiatric nursing. During the course of the year more than 80 applications were received from State registered nurses for admission to the training course organised by the hospital, and requests have been received from other hospitals and organisations for assistance in the training of staff. This indicates not only interest in the subject, but also a realisation of the necessity for adequate training in this special branch of nursing, which calls for a high standard of ability in the nurse and makes perhaps more demands upon her personality and skill than in most other branches of her profession.

At the request of the Editor of the *Nursing Mirror*, a joint article on post-graduate training in psychiatry was written by the Medical Director and Matron, to be included in a series on "Careers for the State Registered Nurse." The article contained many illustrations depicting the life and work of the hospital.

A Cassel Hospital Nurses' League has been formed so that those holding post-graduate certificates may have an opportunity of meeting to discuss and further their knowledge and experience.

The Cassel Bursaries

A short intensive course of four months' duration in contrast with the 18 months required for the full training, has been undertaken during the year. This course, which is reserved for senior members of the nursing profession desiring to gain some insight into psychological medicine, was made possible by the generosity of Sir Felix Cassel. The Bursary students have spent two months working in the wards of the hospital, one month under the auspices of the National Council for Mental Health in London, and a fourth month in the Occupational Therapy department of the hospital. During this time they received an intensive course of lectures from the members of the staff of the hospital.

Thanks must be given to the National Council for Mental Health for their continued co-operation in this experiment which has proved of the greatest value. The range of experience provided for the students has enabled them to gain good insight into the problems of psychiatric nursing.

OCCUPATIONAL THERAPY DEPARTMENT, ENTERTAINMENTS, LIBRARY, ETC.

Occupational Therapist.—Miss M. DAWSON.

In Charge of Library, "Keep Fit" Classes and Country Dancing.—Miss M. STILES (*Physiotherapist*).

In Charge of Gardening Teams.—Mr. G. SNAPE (*Physiotherapist*).

Occupational Therapy

Occupational Therapy at the Cassel Hospital is divided into three main grades. The first may be termed diversional occupational therapy, the second creative, and the third, while being as far as possible creative, is intended to adjust the patient towards his final return to normal life.

Stage 1. This is intended for those patients whose powers of concentration are limited and who have for the moment little capacity for creative work. Most of these patients urgently require to be diverted from their preoccupations with their own symptoms. There is a need at this stage for the achievement of attractive results in a short time with comparatively little technical skill. Cane work which has hitherto been one of the best crafts for this purpose has necessarily been reduced owing to severe shortage of materials. String work, has to some extent taken the place of work with cane, since this too can readily be adapted to the requirements of individual patients and string is still plentiful. Rug making of various types is useful, but materials are expensive and still difficult to obtain. Soft toymaking, stool seating, and sometimes needlework and knitting are also valuable.

Stage 2. When the patients' powers of concentration improve, creative occupational therapy of a more technically difficult kind can be introduced. This serves a wider and more useful purpose than the merely diversional form of activity. Leather work is here especially valuable and can be adjusted in difficulty to suit various needs. Weaving and bookbinding are also valuable, and carpentry is useful for the men. Among the work produced in the carpenter's shop for general use has been a very elaborate model theatre, many toys for the Day Nurseries and equipment for the hospital such as a notice board and apparatus for table tennis, etc.

Stage 3. At this stage we endeavour as far as possible to introduce occupations which take the patient beyond the precincts of the hospital. He is thus brought into closer contact with normal life and with the type of activity which he will have to undertake when he leaves the sheltered environment of the hospital. We have been fortunate in securing the co-operation of certain individuals and firms for this purpose, and it has been possible to send patients to a variety of outside tasks. Included among these are farming, work in a day nursery, work at the W.V.S. depot, canteen work, clerical work and work in a bookshop.

During the course of the year the period of work in the Occupational Therapy Department has been increased by the introduction of an afternoon session at which mainly group activities have been undertaken, such as the repair of hospital linen, etc. Whenever possible, a number of patients work in the garden during the afternoon under the direction of Mr. G. Snape, physiotherapist. These patients have been largely responsible for maintaining the state of cultivation of the grounds. Such work is very appropriately supervised by the physiotherapist, who is able to grade the activities undertaken according to the physical capacity of each of the patients under his care, and is also able to encourage and reassure those who are doubtful about their physical capacity to perform a particular task.

During part of the year working parties were held under the supervision of Miss Stiles to make carpet slippers for hospitals, the materials for which were supplied through the Hanley Red Cross and St. John Organisation. Working parties were started again towards the end of the year in order to make toys for the Christmas tree. The results were excellent and the patients saw the delight of the children as they received the toys.

Students

Students of Occupational Therapy from the Dorset House School worked in the Department throughout the year. Several members of the nursing staff each spent a period in the Occupational Therapy Department learning types of work prescribed for patients and gaining further insight into occupational therapy. The first two Cassel Bursary students also came for one month each to gain some insight into this branch of psychiatric treatment. Lectures on the work were also given by the Occupational Therapist.

Entertainments

As in previous years the patients elected entertainments' committees from among their own number, and with the co-operation of members of the staff devised their weekly entertainments. A notable contribution to these was the construction of a marionette theatre upon which a very successful play was produced under the supervision of Miss Barclay at that time working as a student in the Occupational Therapy Department. It is hoped to develop this form of activity to a considerable extent.

Cinema

Weekly films were given throughout the winter to patients and others. Documentary and feature films were shown alternately and, as always, proved very popular.

Games

Lack of equipment limited outdoor games. A few tennis balls were available for use and croquet and putting were also enjoyed. Table tennis remained the most popular indoor game, several matches being played between patients and staff.

Library

During the course of the year the average number of daily issues from the library increased steadily. The catalogue now contains a very wide range of books, so that it is possible to satisfy almost all tastes.

Through the generosity of the Chairman in making a personal gift to the library, and through a grant made by the Committee, it has been possible to add a number of new books during the year and to increase the range of magazines for which subscriptions are held.

As in previous years the library has been in charge of three patients responsible to the chief librarian. The librarians who have taken a share of duty during the year have done good work, and one subsequently trained under the Red Cross in preparation for library work in one of their hospitals.

A book plate has been designed and is being put into all new books. It depicts a man standing at the gateway of a new life and stepping from darkness into light.

PHYSIOTHERAPY

Physiotherapists : Mr. G. SNAPE, C.S.P., Miss M. STILES, C.S.P.

During the course of the year a Sunlight Apparatus was purchased and has proved valuable for the treatment of patients confined to bed for considerable periods. Massage and graduated exercises have, as always, proved valuable for such patients, particularly those who have suffered from prolonged complaints of fatigue. Some of these patients have been bedridden for months before reaching hospital, and their physical tone has therefore been correspondingly poor. For the women patients there has been a Keep-Fit Class, held twice weekly under the auspices of Miss Stiles, which has been very successful. Country Dancing, which is held weekly during the winter months has also been valuable.

The gardening team under the direction of Mr G. Snape has provided physical rehabilitation for most of the men and some of the women patients.

ANNUAL STATISTICAL TABLES FOR 1944

Results for 1944

One hundred cases were discharged from the Hospital during the year 1944. Of these seven were discharged within one month as being unsuitable for treatment in this hospital. This total is slightly lower than the corresponding one for the year 1943, in which 111 patients were treated. The reduction was due to staff illness and other unavoidable causes which reflect sharply upon the working of a small unit when staff is already at a bare minimum. The waiting list has tended to increase in length and remains a serious problem.

The diagnostic categories in which patients are grouped show little change. Affective Neuroses (anxiety states) show a slight increase and hysterical reactions a decrease. Thus in 1943, 28 per cent. of patients discharged had suffered from affective neurosis and 16 per cent. from hysteria. In 1944 34 per cent. of discharges had suffered from affective neurosis and 9 per cent. from hysteria. Such changes occurring from one year to the next, which are not part of a consistent trend, have little significance.

Follow-up Tables

Considering the many difficulties created by war time changes of address, service overseas, etc., the total number of patients replying to the follow-up letters was very high. Approximately 428 letters were sent out and 272 replies were received. It is natural that for the earlier years the response was less good. Of the 130 patients discharged during 1940 only 49 replied, whereas, of the 111 patients discharged during 1943, 88 replied. It would be dangerous to draw conclusions from the figures for the 1940 patients since the proportion responding is low. It is hoped that, after the war, the services of a trained social worker may be obtained to compare the results of our survey with those which might be obtained by a more complete investigation. From the figures here shown it is possible to state that there has been no change for the worse in the follow-up results compared with earlier years. Neither war conditions, nor the use of shorter time saving methods of treatment have therefore affected our results over the period under review.

TABLE I

Total Number of Patients Discharged from Hospital

during 1944

New Patients	Re-admissions	Total	Discharged unsuitable within one month	Total in which treatment undertaken
89	11	100	7	93

9

TABLE 2   Total Number of Patients for whom Treatment was Undertaken during 1944.   Classification by Diagnosis, Sex and Condition on Discharge

Diagnosis	MALES				FEMALES				TOTALS			
	Much Imp.	Imp.	Not Imp.	Total	Much Imp.	Imp.	Not Imp.	Total	Much Imp.	Imp.	Not Imp.	Total
Affective Neurosis	8	3	—	11	9	8	4	21	17	11	4	32
Hysteria	1	1	—	2	1	5	—	6	2	6	—	8
Anorexia Nervosa	—	—	—	—	2	—	—	2	2	—	—	2
Obsessive Compulsive Neurosis	—	1	—	1	1	2	—	3	1	3	—	4
Psychopathic Personalities ...	—	1	2	3	1	2	3	6	1	3	5	9
Unclassified Neurosis ...	1	1	1	3	1	1	—	2	2	2	1	5
Alcoholism and Drug Addiction	1	—	1	2	—	2	—	2	1	2	1	4
Affective Psychosis (depression)	11	—	—	11	8	4	—	12	19	4	—	23
Schizophrenic and Paranoid Reaction	—	—	2	2	—	—	1	1	—	—	3	3
Organic and Toxic Reaction	—	1	—	1	—	2	—	2	—	3	—	3
Total	22	8	6	36	23	26	8	57	45	34	14	93
Percentage	61%	22%	17%	100%	40%	46%	14%	100%	48%	37%	15%	100%

TABLE 3   Percentage Distribution of Results on Discharge and at Follow-up

(a) Cases Discharged during 1940

Condition	On Discharge	Follow-up			
		1941	1942	1943	1944
Much improved ...	42	44	49	56	53
Improved	40	27	24	19	6
Not Improved ...	18	29	27	25	41*
Total ...	100	100	100	100	100
Total cases on which percentage based...	130	68	66	48	49
Number not replying to follow-up ...	—	62	64	82	81

* Including 18% (9 cases) dead.

(b) Cases Discharged during 1941

Condition	On Discharge	Follow-up		
		1942	1943	1944
Much Improved ...	52	54	50	41
Improved	34	19	23	18
Not Improved ...	14	27	27	41*
Total	100	100	100	100
Total cases on which percentage based...	85	59	52	54
Number not replying to follow-up ...	—	26	33	31

* Including 11% (6 cases) dead.

(c) Cases Discharged during 1942

Condition	On Discharge	Follow-up	
		1943	1944
Much Improved ...	55	62	57
Improved ...	27	20	17
Not Improved	18	18	26*
Total	100	100	100
Total cases on which percentage based ...	102	81	81
Number not replying to follow-up	—	21	21

* Including 5% (4 cases) dead.

(d) Cases Discharged during 1943

Condition	On Discharge	Follow-up 1944
Much Improved	50	42
Improved	31	31
Not Improved	19	27*
Total	100	100
Total cases on which percentage based	111	88
Number not replying to follow-up ...	—	23

* Including 7% (6 cases) dead.

Report of the General Committee

GENERAL

Committee Members

THE Committee has to record with great pleasure that a Peerage was conferred by His Majesty on Sir Courtauld-Thomson, K.B.E., C.B., on the 1st January, 1944. The Lord Courtauld-Thomson, K.B.E., C.B., has been a member of the Committee since the foundation of the hospital and is one of the Trustees. The Committee desire to express to him their warmest congratulations on this honour which has been so fully earned by many years of public and philanthropic service.

During the year the Committee has suffered sad losses by the deaths of three most valuable members.

Mrs. E. JOSHUA, who died on 11th June, 1944, had been a member of the General Committee since 1919 and had rendered most valuable service, more particularly in connection with domestic matters.

Miss WINIFRED THOMSON, who died on 15th August, 1944, had been a member of the General Committee since 1933. She had always been most kind and helpful, especially in advising on domestic matters relating to the hospital and she will be sadly missed.

Sir ARTHUR HURST, who died on 17th August, 1944, had been a member of the General and Medical Committees since the foundation of the hospital and had always taken a great interest in its work. It was his work at Seale Hayne during the last war that influenced the founder, Sir Ernest Cassel, in his decision to endow a hospital for functional nervous disorders. Sir Arthur's help and advice were always at the disposal of the hospital when there was any particular problem to meet and his death was a very great loss.

A further loss to the Committee occurred in July 1944 when Lady Helen Cassel was compelled to resign owing to ill health. Lady Helen had been a member of the General Committee since 1927. She played a very active part in the affairs of the hospital, particularly in connection with domestic and nursing matters and served on many sub-committees. The Committee desires to extend to her its sympathy and good wishes.

In July 1944 the Committee welcomed Mrs. Pugh as a new member to the General Committee.

Committee Visits

On 28th April, 1944, Lady Louis Mountbatten visited the hospital while making a tour in North Staffordshire in connection with her work as Superintendent-in-Chief of the St. John Ambulance Brigade. She inspected the hospital premises, saw the work which was being carried out and talked with many of the staff and patients.

On 27th May, 1944, Air-Commodore R. D. Gillespie, M.D., F.R.C.P., paid a visit to the hospital. He distributed certificates to the sisters who had completed the course of training in psychological nursing and gave the prizes for essays written in connection with their final examination. A large audience witnessed the prize-giving, among them doctors and nurses from neighbouring hospitals and representatives of allied fields of social service. Lectures were given by Dr. Andratschke the Assistant Physician, and also the Matron, and after tea in the lounge there were demonstrations of various methods of treatment used in the hospital, occupational therapy, etc.

Affiliation

Negotiations have been in progress since February 1944 with the governors of Guy's Hospital, for mutual professional collaboration in the post-war period. It has been felt by both parties that the facilities of the department of psychological medicine at the York Clinic at Guy's Hospital and those of the Cassel Hospital when it is re-established at Swaylands, are mutually complementary. It is also felt that the closer association likely to result between the Cassel Hospital and a large general teaching hospital will be beneficial to the advancement of knowledge in the field of psychological medicine.

ASH HALL

Lease

In view of the uncertainty about the probable date of the return to Swaylands, which had not been settled by the end of the year, it was decided to renew the lease of Ash Hall for a further period of two years from 9th November, 1944, with a further option for a third year at the end of this period if it was found desirable.

Waiting List

The small number of beds available at Ash Hall has again resulted in a long waiting list which constitutes a difficult and unsatisfactory problem. The demand for accommodation at the hospital greatly exceeds the available facilities. Admissions have, as far as possible, been limited to those cases for whom the treatment available in the hospital is likely to produce the maximum benefit. From such applicants a priority list has been governed by three main considerations :—

1. Urgency of the medical problem.
2. Importance of the individual to the national war effort.
3. Age of the individual.

No system of selection or of priority, however, will solve the main problem, which is essentially that of inadequacy of facilities for the treatment of neurosis in the country as a whole.

Miscellaneous

Sun Lamp. An " Hanovia " Sun Lamp was purchased in February 1944 to be used for the patients and the staff.

Ford Van. In the summer the hospital Ford Van was re-conditioned throughout. This van, already some seven years old should now give good service for several more years.

Library. The Committee made a grant for 1944 for the purchase of library books. This was supplemented by a generous gift from the Chairman. As a result it was possible to add 30 new volumes to the library and to increase the range of subscriptions to magazines of general interest.

Staff

The senior permanent staff remained the same as in 1943, with the exception of Miss Dawson, who left in November 1944 to organise occupational therapy in government hospitals in New Zealand. Miss M. P. R. Barclay was appointed as Occupational Therapist in Miss Dawson's stead, to commence in 1945.

Hospital Badge. A hospital badge was designed and introduced for members of the nursing staff who had completed their period of training for the hospital certificate. The badge bears the motto " Lux ex tenebris."

Recreational Facilities. In April 1944, the Committee made a grant for the purpose of increasing recreational and cultural amenities for the staff. A hall was hired for badminton and during the winter months lectures were arranged through the Workers' Educational Association.

At the close of another year of successful work the Committee desires to express its appreciation to the staff of the hospital for their continued zeal and ability under the many difficulties imposed on an evacuated unit. Knowing that many are far away from home, the Committee hopes that it may not be long before they are able to return to familiar quarters.

SWAYLANDS

Architect

The Committee has to record with regret the death of Mr. J. Maclaren Ross, A.R.I.B.A., which occurred on 2nd March, 1944. Mr. Ross, who was the brother of the late Dr. T. A. Ross, had been architect to the hospital for 20 years. He had always taken such a detailed interest in the buildings that he will be much missed.

Messrs. Young & Hall, of Southampton Row, W.C.1, were chosen by the Committee in July 1944 to prepare plans, etc. in connection with the return to Swaylands of the hospital unit after the war. Meetings and preliminary discussions of the problems to be solved have already been held.

De-Requisitioning of Swaylands

In November 1944, the War Office was approached regarding the possibility of the de-requisitioning of Swaylands. A reply was received saying that the hospital was being used to meet important military requirements and that no date could yet be foreseen when the building could be de-requisitioned. Since the end of the year at the request of the Committee, the Ministry of Health have made strong representations to the War Department with a view to hastening the de-requisitioning.

War Damage

Some staff cottages and farm buildings sustained small amounts of damage from bomb blast during the year. Repair work was done by our local contractors and a claim has been lodged with the War Damage Commission.

Wives and families of some of the gardeners left the district during the V.1 bombing period, July 1944, but quickly returned when conditions became more normal.

Cottages

The cottages previously occupied by doctors and secretary continue to be let satisfactorily.

Engineer and Carpenter

The engineer, Mr. W. Finkle, and the carpenter Mr. C. Cole, at present employed by the military authorities, have given much help in their spare time with problems which have arisen in connection with the premises at Swaylands.

SWAYLANDS GARDENS

Honey Field

A field of seven acres known as the " Honey Field," previously let for grazing, was put under the plough in the autumn in order to provide more extensive and more economical cultivation. A government grant for this additional ploughed land has been received.

Implements

The purchase of a re-conditioned Fordson Tractor and a Robot Transplanter have proved of great help in running the gardens on a market garden basis.

Vegetables and Fruit

As in previous years, weekly supplies of vegetables and fruit in season have been sent up to Ash Hall through the kind assistance of the Southern Railway, who also arranged transport in the autumn of pickled eggs, jam and bottled fruit, which had been prepared for the hospital by the head gardener's wife, Mrs. Herbert.

Although the gardens do not show such a good surplus as for last year, owing to bad weather at planting time, severe late frosts which reduced drastically the amount of fruit and necessary expenditure on equipment, the results are better than were expected.

The Committee desires to place on record its continued appreciation of the excellent work done by the head gardener and his staff.

FINANCE

The Accounts for the year ended 31st December, 1944, show a surplus of Income over Expenditure of £2,624 compared with £3,819 in the previous year. This surplus is almost entirely due to the rent received for Swaylands, and it may be that the surplus arising from this cause during the war will be insufficient to meet the heavy outlay which will have to be incurred in connection with the return to Swaylands to which reference is made below. During the year appreciable rises in costs occurred, due mainly to the higher rates of pay to the Nursing and Domestic staff in accordance with the recommendations of the Rushcliffe and Hetherington Reports. Other contributory factors to the higher expenditure were increased fuel and domestic costs and, to a lesser degree, the purchase of a small quantity of electrical apparatus for special treatments. These rising costs are entirely outside the control of the Committee, who in order to avoid incurring a deficit on the working of the Hospital have found it necessary to make a small increase in the rate of fees charged to patients. From July 1944, these were adjusted to give a weekly average of £6 10s. per patient. As a result, the total fees

for the year are substantially the same as in the previous year, in spite of a reduction in the average number of patients from 29.21 to 27.28 per day.

There was a surplus of Extraordinary Income over Extraordinary Expenditure of £2,535 compared with £2,765 a year ago. Market gardening at Swaylands resulted in a surplus of £41 compared with £771 a year ago. This reduction is largely attributable to the cost of replacing the tractor and the purchase of a robot transplanter ; in addition, late frosts and adverse weather conditions were responsible for reduced crops.

In accordance with the policy adopted in recent years the whole of the surplus of Income over Expenditure has been earmarked for the reinstatement of the Hospital at Swaylands. Alternative schemes for the reinstatement of the Hospital have been examined and estimates of the maintenance costs likely to be incurred at Swaylands have been prepared. From these it is apparent that it will no longer be possible to conduct the Hospital as an economic unit on lines similar to those in force before the war. To take just one example, the recruitment of the large staff of domestic servants required in the existing buildings had already become extremely difficult before the war and, apart from the fact that it may be impossible in the post-war era to obtain the necessary domestic staff, the changed rates of pay and conditions of employment are such as to become a disproportionate expense to the normal maintenance of a patient. This can only be avoided by drastic structural alterations or by entirely rebuilding the Hospital, either of which may be impractical for some years to come. The temporary war-time reduction in the number of patients from 64 to 30 has lessened the normal renewals of bedding, linen, crockery, etc., so that as soon as the numbers are once again increased, considerable expenditure will be needed even to bring the supplies up to the minimum establishment requirements. These facts should therefore be taken into account when considering the surplus revenue shown by the Accounts in recent years, and the sum necessarily earmarked for the reinstatement of the Hospital.

During the year the only changes in the Investments have been the purchase of £3,500 2½ per cent. Funding Loan 1956/61 and the redemption at par of a further £100 Irish Free State 4½ per cent. Land Bonds. The total book value of the Investments at 31st December, 1944 was £147,655 5s. 8d. (compared with £144,366 11s. 8d. a year ago), the market valuation being £154,558 7s. 4d., or £6,903 1s. 8d. in excess of the book value.

INCOME AND EXPENDITURE ACCOUNT FOR THE YEAR ENDED 31st DECEMBER, 1944

INCOME

	£ s. d.	£ s. d.
Ordinary—		
I. Receipts on Account of Services Rendered		
From Patients—		
Fees	9,344 4 6	
II. Invested Property Interest, Dividends, etc. ...	5,349 11 11	
Ordinary Income ...		14,693 16 5
Extraordinary—		
I. Rents of Evacuated Properties ...	2,987 12 4	
II. Surplus on Swaylands Gardens ...	41 2 6	
Extraordinary Income		3,028 14 10
TOTAL INCOME		£17,722 11 3

EXPENDITURE

	£ s. d.	£ s. d.
Ordinary—		
I. Provisions		1,825 17 2
II. Surgery and Dispensary ...		368 15 4
III. Domestic		1,543 13 2
IV. Salaries and Wages (Maintenance)		7,870 2 0
V. Miscellaneous		792 5 9
VI. Administration		1,120 4 3
VII. Establishment		74 18 10
VIII. Finance		1,008 5 9
Ordinary Expenditure		14,604 2 3
Extraordinary—		
I. Upkeep of Evacuated Properties (including War Damage Insurance)	494 2 1	
Extraordinary Expenditure		494 2 1
TOTAL EXPENDITURE		15,098 4 4
Balance, being excess of Total Income over Total Expenditure for the year		2,624 6 11
		£17,722 11 3

BALANCE SHEET, 31st DECEMBER, 1944

	£ s. d.	£ s. d.	£ s. d.
Creditors—			
Tradesmen's Accounts and Accrued Expenses ...			1,330 19 3
Capital Accounts—			
(a) Founder's Trust Fund as at 31st December, 1943 ...		220,532 0 0	
Less: Loss on Redemption of Investment ...		10 8 0	
		220,521 12 0	
(b) Special Funds as at 31st December 1943—			
THE KATHARINE WALEY COHEN TRUST FUND—gift for special purposes	1,682 1 6		
THE H.G.K. TRUST FUND—gift for special purposes	500 0 0		
THE BERNARD TEMPLE WRINCH SETTLEMENT—bequest for general purposes	7,782 13 0		
THE MARY ANN OAKE BEQUEST	597 19 6		
		10,462 14 0	
(c) General Fund as at 31st December, 1943 ... 24,766 0 10			
Add: Excess of Income over Expenditure for the year ended 31st December, 1944, per annexed Account	2,624 6 11		
		27,390 7 9	
			268,874 13 9
Unexpended Income Balance of Special Fund—			
Medical Director's Special Fund as at 31st December, 1943	124 19 7		
Add: Interest and Donations for year ...	401 3 1		
	526 2 8		
Less Grants during year ...	113 4 0		
			412 18 8
			£260,418 11 8

NOTE.—The General Fund is earmarked for the reinstatement of the Hospital at Swaylands.

	£ s. d.	£ s. d.	£ s. d.
Cash at Bank and in Hand—On Account of—			
(1) General Fund ...		2,452 16 5	
(2) Medical Director's Special Fund ...		412 18 8	
			2,865 15 1
Stocks on Hand ...			568 5 5
Debtors and Payments in Advance ...			589 17 4
Interest Accrued on Investments ...			1,858 17 6
Investments at Cost—			
(a) Founder's Trust Fund ...		113,941 1 4	
(b) Special Funds—			
THE KATHARINE WALEY COHEN TRUST FUND ...	1,682 1 6		
THE H.G.K. TRUST FUND ...	500 0 0		
THE BERNARD TEMPLE WRINCH SETTLEMENT ...	7,782 13 0		
THE MARY ANN OAKE BEQUEST ...	597 19 6		
		10,462 14 0	
(c) General Fund (Market Value £154,558 7 4½)		23,251 10 4	
			147,655 5 8
Land, Buildings and Equipment—			
As at 31st December, 1943 ...			106,880 10 8
			£260,418 11 8

We have audited the above Balance Sheet dated 31st December, 1944, and have obtained all the information and explanations we have required. In our opinion such Balance Sheet is properly drawn up so as to exhibit a true and correct view of the state of affairs, according to the best of our information and the explanations given to us and as shown by the books of the Hospital.

BARTON, MAYHEW & CO.,
Chartered Accountants.

ALDERMAN'S HOUSE, BISHOPSGATE,
LONDON, E.C.2.
26th July, 1945.

INVESTMENTS AT COST—AS AT 31st DECEMBER, 1944

	£ s. d.	£ s. d.
(a) Founders' Trust Fund—		
£3,237/13/6 3½% Conversion Loan, 1961	2,476 19 7	
£3,500 2½% Funding Loan, 1956/61	3,399 2 0	
£2,000 2½% National War Bonds 1945/47	2,021 5 4	
£33,200 3% Savings Bonds 1955/65 " B "	33,205 15 9	
£8,900 3% Savings Bonds 1955/65	8,900 0 0	
£8,200 3% Savings Bonds 1960/70 " A "	8,200 0 0	
£900 3% Defence Bonds P.O. 3rd Issue	900 0 0	
£9,676/15/7 3½% War Loan	9,547 16 4	
£15,500 Local Loans 3% Stock	12,702 9 6	
£10,000 Birmingham Corporation 4½% Redeemable Stock, 1945/55 ...	9,853 15 0	
£1,500 Bristol Corporation 3% Loan 1958/63	1,491 12 3	
£500 London Transport 5% "A" Stock	496 18 0	
£2,000 London Transport 5% " B " Stock	2,279 11 0	
£5,796/9/7 Commonwealth of Australia 5% Registered Stock, 1945/75	5,711 13 8	
£7,200 London & North Eastern Railway 4% 1st Preference Stock ...	4,973 8 9	
£3,000 Barclay Perkins & Co., Ltd., 3½% Mortgage Debenture Stock	3,020 0 3	
£3,100 Bass Ratcliff & Gretton Ltd., 3½% "B" Mortgage Debenture Stock	3,153 14 9	
£368 William Younger & Co. Ltd. 3½% Debenture Stock ...	333 18 4	
£1,150 South Suburban Gas Co., 5% Perpetual Debenture Stock ...	1,273 0 10	
(Market Value £117,713 19 9)		113,941 1 4
(b) Special Funds—		
THE KATHARINE WALEY COHEN TRUST FUND—		
£1,665 Shell Transport & Trading Co., Limited, 5% 1st Preference Stock. Fully paid (Market Value £2,206 2 6)	1,582 1 6	
THE H.G.K. TRUST FUND—		
£496/4/6 3½% War Loan (Market Value £516 13 10)	500 0 0	
THE BERNARD TEMPLE WRINCH SETTLEMENT—		
£7,807/6/0 Consolidated 4% Stock (Market Value £8,588 0 7)	7,782 13 0	
THE MARY ANN OAKE BEQUEST—		
£100 3% Defence Bonds. P.O. Issue 100 0 0		
£495/17/5 3½% War Loan 497 19 6		
£250 Textile Trades Corporation Berlin 7% Stock Trust Certificates... ... ... —		
(Market Value £616 6 6)	597 19 6	
		10,462 14 0
(c) General Fund—		
£153/13/5 3½% War Loan	151 12 5	
£7,222/19/6 Consolidated 4% Stock	7,200 4 0	
£14,114 Irish Free State 4½% Land Bonds	15,581 15 5	
£335 Shell Transport and Trading Co., Ltd., 5% 1st Preference Stock. Fully paid	317 18 6	
(Market Value £24,917 4 2)		23,251 10 4
		£147,655 5 8

STATISTICAL TABLES FOR THE YEAR ENDED 31st DECEMBER, 1944
and comparison with the Year ended 31st December, 1943

ACCOMMODATION	1944	1943
Number of available beds	30	30
Average number of patients resident daily	27.28	29.21
Number of admissions during the year	102	113
Number of discharges during the year	101	116
Number remaining at 31st December	28	27

EXPENDITURE	Expenditure for the year ended 31st Dec., 1944	Average weekly cost per patient during 1944	1943
ORDINARY	£ s. d.	£ s. d.	£ s. d.
Provisions	1,825 17 2	1 5 9	1 5 9
Surgery and Dispensary	368 15 4	5 2	2 11
Domestic	1,543 13 2	1 1 8	16 9
Salaries and Wages	7,870 2 0	5 10 4	4 14 5
Miscellaneous	792 5 9	11 1	9 6
Administration	1,120 4 3	15 8	14 1
Establishment	74 18 10	1 0	11
Finance	1,008 5 9	14 2	13 5
	14,604 2 3	10 4 10	8 17 9
EXTRAORDINARY	494 2 1	6 11	17 2
Total Cost ...	£15 098 4 4	£10 11 9	£9 14 11